# The Ultimate Mediterranean Cookbook

Get In Shape And Lose Weight With Tasty And Affordable Mediterranean Recipes For Beginners

Dan Peterson

# TABLE OF CONTENT

result of the use of information contained within this document, including, but not limited to, — errors, omissions, or inaccuracies.

# Balsamic Eggplant Mix

Preparation time: 10 minutes
Cooking time : 20 minutes

Servings : 6

INGREDIENTS:
- 1/3 cup chicken stock
- 2 tablespoons balsamic vinegar
- A pinch of salt and black pepper
- 1 tablespoon lime juice
- 2 big eggplants, sliced
- 1 tablespoon rosemary, chopped
- ¼ cup cilantro, chopped
- 2 tablespoons olive oil

DIRECTIONS:
1. In a roasting pan, combine the eggplants with the stock, the vinegar and the rest of the ingredients, introduce the pan in the oven and bake at 390 degrees F for 20 minutes. Divide the mix between plates and serve as a side dish.

NUTRITION: Calories 201 Fat 4.5g Carbs 5.4g Protein 3g

# Sage Barley Mix

Preparation time: 10 minutes
Cooking time : 45 minutes

Servings: 4

INGREDIENTS:
- 1 tablespoon olive oil
- 1 red onion, chopped
- 1 tablespoon leaves, chopped
- 1 garlic clove, minced
- 14 ounces barley
- ½ tablespoon parmesan, grated
- 6 cups veggie stock
- Salt and black pepper to the taste

DIRECTIONS:
1. Heat up a pan with the oil over medium heat, add the onion and garlic, stir and sauté for 5 minutes.
2. Add the sage, barley and the rest of the ingredients except the parmesan, stir, bring to a simmer and cook for 40 minutes. Add the parmesan, stir, divide between plates.

NUTRITION: Calories 210 Fat 6.5g Carbs 8.6g Protein 3.4g

# Chickpeas and Beets Mix

Preparation time: 10 minutes
Cooking time : 25 minutes

Servings: 4

INGREDIENTS:
- 3 tablespoons capers, drained and chopped
- Juice of 1 lemon
- Zest of 1 lemon, grated
- 1 red onion, chopped
- 3 tablespoons olive oil
- 14 ounces canned chickpeas, drained
- 8 ounces beets, peeled and cubed
- 1 tablespoon parsley, chopped
- Salt and pepper to the taste

DIRECTIONS:
1. Heat up a pan with the oil over medium heat, add the onion, lemon zest, lemon juice and the capers and sauté for 5 minutes.
2. Add the rest of the ingredients, stir and cook over medium-low heat for 20 minutes more. Divide the mix between plates and serve as a side dish.

NUTRITION: Calories 199 Fat 4.5g Carbs 6.5g Protein 3.3g

# Creamy Sweet Potatoes Mix

Preparation time:  10 minutes

Cooking time: 1 hour

Servings: 4

INGREDIENTS:
- 4 tablespoons olive oil
- 1 garlic clove, minced
- 4 medium sweet potatoes, pricked with a fork
- 1 red onion, sliced
- 3 ounces baby spinach
- Zest and juice of 1 lemon
- A small bunch dill, chopped
- 1 and ½ tablespoons Greek yogurt
- 2 tablespoons tahini paste
- Salt and black pepper to the taste

DIRECTIONS:
1. Put the potatoes on a baking sheet lined with parchment paper, introduce in the oven at 350 degrees F and cook them for 1 hour.
2. Peel the potatoes, cut them into wedges and put them in a bowl. Add the garlic, the oil and the rest of the ingredients, toss, divide the mix between plates and serve.

NUTRITION: Calories 214 Fat 5.6g Carbs 6.5g Protein 3.1g

# Pasta e Fagioli with Orange and Fennel

Preparation Time: 10 minutes

Cooking Time: 30 minutes

Servings: 5

INGREDIENTS

- Extra-virgin olive oil – 1 tbsp. plus extra for serving
- Pancetta – 2 ounces, chopped fine
- Onion – 1, chopped fine
- Fennel – 1 bulb, stalks discarded, bulb halved, cored, and chopped fine
- Celery – 1 rib, minced
- Garlic – 2 cloves, minced
- Anchovy fillets – 3, rinsed and minced
- Minced fresh oregano – 1 tbsp.
- Grated orange zest – 2 tsp.
- Fennel seeds – ½ tsp.
- Red pepper flakes – ¼ tsp.
- Diced tomatoes – 1 (28-ounce) can
- Parmesan cheese – 1 rind, plus more for serving
- Cannellini beans – 1 (7-ounce) cans, rinsed
- Chicken broth – 2 ½ cups
- Water – 2 ½ cups
- Salt and pepper
- Orzo – 1 cup
- Minced fresh parsley – ¼ cup

DIRECTIONS

1. Heat oil in a Dutch oven over medium heat. Add pancetta.

2. Stir-fry for 3 to 5 minutes or until beginning to brown.
3. Stir in celery, fennel, and onion and stir-fry until softened (about 5 to 7 minutes).
4. Stir in pepper flakes, fennel seeds, orange zest, oregano, anchovies, and garlic. Cook for 1 minute.
5. Stir in tomatoes and their juice. Stir in Parmesan rind and beans.
6. Bring to a simmer and cook for 10 minutes.
7. Stir in water, broth, and 1 tsp. salt.
8. Increase heat to high and bring to a boil.
9. Stir in pasta and cook for 10 minutes, or until al dente.
10. Remove from heat and discard parmesan rind.
11. Stir in parsley and season with salt and pepper to taste.
12. Drizzle with olive oil and sprinkle with grated Parmesan.
13. Serve.

NUTRITION: Calories: 502 Fat: 8.8g Carb: 72.2g Protein: 34.9g

# Spaghetti al Limone

Preparation Time: 10 minutes

Cooking Time: 15 minutes

Servings: 2

INGREDIENTS
- Extra-virgin olive oil – ½ cup
- Grated lemon zest – 2 tsp.
- Lemon juice – 1/3 cup
- Garlic – 1 clove, minced to pate
- Salt and pepper
- Parmesan cheese – 2 ounces, grated
- Spaghetti – 1 pound
- Shredded fresh basil – 6 tbsp.

DIRECTIONS
1. In a bowl, whisk garlic, oil, lemon zest, juice, ½ tsp. salt and ¼ tsp. pepper. Stir in the Parmesan and mix until creamy.
2. Meanwhile, cook the pasta according to package directions. Drain and reserve ½ cup cooking water.
3. Add the oil mixture and basil to the pasta and toss to combine.
4. Season with salt and pepper to taste and add the cooking water as needed.
5. Serve.

NUTRITION: Calories: 398 Fat: 20.7g Carb: 42.5g Protein: 11.9g

# Spiced Vegetable Couscous

Preparation Time: 10 minutes

Cooking Time: 20 minutes

Servings: 2

INGREDIENTS
- Cauliflower – 1 head, cut into 1 –inch florets
- Extra-virgin olive oil – 6 tbsp. plus extra for serving
- Salt and pepper
- Couscous – 1 ½ cups
- Zucchini – 1, cut into ½ inch pieces
- Red bell pepper – 1, stemmed, seeded, and cut into ½ inch pieces
- Garlic – 4 cloves, minced
- Ras el hanout – 2 tsp.
- Grated lemon zest -1 tsp. plus lemon wedges for serving
- Chicken broth – 1 ¾ cups
- Minced fresh marjoram – 1 tbsp.

DIRECTIONS
1. In a skillet, heat 2 tbsp. oil over medium heat.
2. Add cauliflowers, ¾ tsp. salt, and ½ tsp. pepper. Mix.
3. Cover and cook for 5 minutes, or until the florets start to brown and the edges are just translucent.
4. Remove the lid and cook, stirring for 10 minutes, or until the florets turn golden

brown. Transfer to a bowl and clean the skillet.

5. Heat 2 tbsp. oil in the skillet.
6. Add the couscous. Cook and stir for 3 to 5 minutes, or until grains are just beginning to brown. Transfer to a bowl and clean the skillet.
7. Heat the remaining 3 tbsp. oil in the skillet and add bell pepper, zucchini, and ½ tsp. salt. Cook for 6 to 8 minutes, or until tender.
8. Stir in lemon zest, ras el hanout, and garlic. Cook until fragrant (about 30 seconds).
9. Stir in the broth and bring to a simmer.
10. Stir in the couscous. Cover, remove from the heat, and set aside until tender (about 7 minutes).
11. Add marjoram and cauliflower; then gently fluff with a fork to combine.
12. Drizzle with extra oil and season with salt and pepper.
13. Serve with lemon wedges.

NUTRITION: Calories: 787 Fat: 18.3g Carb: 129.6g Protein: 24.5g

# Spiced Baked Rice with Fennel

Preparation Time: 10 minutes

Cooking Time: 45 minutes

Servings: 2

INGREDIENTS
- Sweet potatoes – 1 ½ pounds, peeled and cut into 1-inch pieces
- Extra-virgin olive oil – ¼ cup
- Salt and pepper
- Fennel – 1 bulb, chopped fine
- Small onion – 1, chopped fine
- Long-grain white rice – 1 ½ cups, rinsed
- Garlic – 4 cloves, minced
- Ras el hanout – 2 tsp.
- Chicken broth – 2 ¾ cups
- Large pitted brine-cured green olives – ¾ cup, halved
- Minced fresh cilantro – 2 tbsp.
- Lime wedges

DIRECTIONS
1. Adjust the oven rack to the middle position and heat the oven to 400F. Toss the potatoes with ½ tsp. salt and 2 tbsp. oil.
2. Arrange the potatoes in a single layer in a rimmed baking sheet and roast for 25 to 30 minutes, or until tender. Stir the potatoes halfway through roasting.
3. Remove the potatoes from the oven and lower the oven temperature to 350F.

4. In a Dutch oven, heat the remaining 2 tbsp. oil over medium heat.
5. Add onion and fennel; next, cook for 5 to 7 minutes, or until softened. Stir in ras el hanout, garlic, and rice. Stir-fry for 3 minutes.
6. Stir in the olives and broth and let sit for 10 minutes. Add the potatoes to the rice and fluff gently with a fork to combine.
7. Season with salt and pepper to taste.
8. Sprinkle with cilantro and serve with lime wedges.

NUTRITION: Calories: 207 Fat: 8.9g Carb: 29.4g Protein: 3.9g

# Moroccan-Style Couscous with Chickpeas

Preparation Time: 5 minutes

Cooking Time: 18 minutes

Servings: 2

INGREDIENTS
- Extra-virgin olive oil – ¼ cup, extra for serving
- Couscous – 1 ½ cups
- Peeled and chopped fine carrots – 2
- Chopped fine onion – 1
- Salt and pepper
- Garlic – 3 cloves, minced
- Ground coriander – 1 tsp.
- Ground ginger - tsp.
- Ground anise seed – ¼ tsp.
- Chicken broth – 1 ¾ cups
- Chickpeas - 1 (15-ounce) can, rinsed
- Frozen peas – 1 ½ cups
- Chopped fresh parsley or cilantro – ½ cup
- Lemon wedges

DIRECTIONS
1. Heat 2 tbsp. oil in a skillet over medium heat.
2. Add the couscous and cook for 3 to 5 minutes, or until just beginning to brown.
3. Transfer to a bowl and clean the skillet.
4. Heat remaining 2 tbsp. oil in the skillet and add the onion, carrots, and 1 tsp. salt.
5. Cook for 5 to 7 minutes, or until softened.

6. Stir in anise, ginger, coriander, and garlic. Cook until fragrant (about 30 seconds).
7. Stir in the chickpeas and broth and bring to simmer.
8. Stir in the couscous and peas. Cover and remove from the heat. Set aside for 7 minutes, or until the couscous is tender.
9. Add the parsley to the couscous and fluff with a fork to combine.
10. Drizzle with extra oil and season with salt and pepper.
11. Serve with lemon wedges.

NUTRITION: Calories: 649 Fat: 14.2g Carb: 102.8g Protein: 30.1g

# Vegetarian Paella with Green Beans and Chickpeas

Preparation Time: 10 minutes

Cooking Time: 35 minutes

Servings: 2

INGREDIENTS
- Pinch of saffron
- Vegetable broth – 3 cups
- Olive oil – 1 tbsp.
- Yellow onion – 1 large, diced
- Garlic – 4 cloves, sliced
- Red bell pepper – 1, diced
- Crushed tomatoes – ¾ cup, fresh or canned
- Tomato paste – 2 tbsp.
- Hot paprika – 1 ½ tsp.
- Salt – 1 tsp.
- Freshly ground black pepper – ½ tsp.
- Green beans – 1 ½ cups, trimmed and halved
- Chickpeas – 1 (15-ounce) can, drained and rinsed
- Short-grain white rice – 1 cup
- Lemon – 1, cut into wedges

DIRECTIONS
1. Mix the saffron threads with 3 tbsp. warm water in a small bowl.
2. In a saucepan, bring the water to a simmer over medium heat. Lower the heat to low

and let the broth simmer.
3. Heat the oil in a skillet over medium heat. Add the onion and stir-fry for 5 minutes.
4. Add the bell pepper and garlic and stir-fry for 7 minutes or until pepper is softened.
5. Stir in the saffron-water mixture, salt, pepper, paprika, tomato paste, and tomatoes.
6. Add the rice, chickpeas, and green beans. Add the warm broth and bring to a boil.
7. Lower the heat and simmer uncovered for 20 minutes.
8. Serve hot, garnished with lemon wedges.

NUTRITION: Calories: 709 Fat: 12g Carb: 121g Protein: 33g

# Garlic Prawns with Tomatoes and Basil

Preparation Time: 10 minutes

Cooking Time: 10 minutes

Servings: 2

INGREDIENTS
- Olive oil – 2 tbsp.
- Prawns – 1 ¼ pounds, peeled and deveined
- Garlic – 3 cloves, minced
- Crushed red pepper flakes – 1/8 tsp.
- Dry white wine – ¾ cup
- Grape tomatoes – 1 ½ cups
- Finely chopped fresh basil – ¼ cup, plus more for garnish
- Salt – ¾ tsp.
- Ground black pepper – ½ tsp.

DIRECTIONS
1. In a skillet, heat oil over medium-high heat. Add the prawns and cook for 1 minute, or until just cooked through. Transfer to a plate.
2. Add the red pepper flakes, and garlic to the oil in the pan and cook, stirring, for 30 seconds. Stir in the wine and cook until it's reduced by about half.
3. Add the tomatoes and stir-fry until tomatoes begin to break down (about 3 to 4 minutes). Stir in the reserved shrimp, salt, pepper, and basil. Cook for 1 to 2 minutes more.
4. Serve garnished with the remaining basil.

NUTRITION: Calories: 282 Fat: 10g Carb: 7g
Protein: 33g

# Stuffed Calamari in Tomato Sauce

Preparation Time: 10 minutes

Cooking Time: 25 minutes

Servings: 2

INGREDIENTS
- Olive oil – ½ cup, plus 3 tbsp. divided
- Large onions - 2, finely chopped
- Garlic – 4 cloves, finely chopped
- Grated Pecorino Romano – 1 cup, plus ¼ cup, divided
- Chopped flat-leaf parsley – ½ cup, plus ¼ cup, divided
- Breadcrumbs – 6 cups
- Raisins – 1 cup
- Large squid tubes – 12, cleaned
- Toothpicks – 12
- For the tomato sauce
- Olive oil – 2 tbsp.
- Garlic – 4 cloves, chopped
- Crushed tomatoes – 2 (28-ounce) cans
- Finely chopped basil – ½ cup
- Salt – 1 tsp.
- Pepper – 1 tsp.

DIRECTIONS
1. Combine the saffron threads with 2 tbsp. of warm water.
2. In a Dutch oven, heat ½ cup of olive oil. Add the onions and ½ tsp. of salt and stir-fry for 5 minutes. Add the tomato paste and cook for 1 minute more.

3. Add the wine and bring to a boil. Add the fish broth and soaked saffron and bring back to a boil. Lower the heat to low and simmer, uncovered, for 10 minutes.
4. Meanwhile, in a food processor, combine the bread and garlic, and process until ground.
5. Add the remaining ¼ cup olive oil and ½ tsp. salt and pulse just to mix.
6. Add the fish to the pot, cover, and cook until the fish is just cooked through, about 6 minutes. Stir in the sauce. Taste and adjust the seasoning.
7. Ladle the stew into the serving bowls.
8. Serve garnished with parsley.

NUTRITION: Calories: 779 Fat: 41g Carb: 31g Protein: 67g

# Provencal Braised Hake

Preparation Time: 10 minutes

Cooking Time: 20 minutes

Servings: 2

INGREDIENTS
- Extra-virgin olive oil – 2 tbsp. plus extra for serving
- Onion – 1, halved and sliced thin
- Fennel bulb – 1, stalks discarded, bulb halved, cored and sliced thin
- Salt and black pepper
- Garlic clove – 4, minced
- Minced fresh thyme – 1 tsp.
- Diced tomatoes – 1 (14.5 ounce) can, drained
- Dry white wine – ½ cup
- Skinless hake fillets – 4 (4 to 6 ounce) 1 to 1 ½ inches thick
- Minced fresh parsley – 2 Tbsp.

DIRECTIONS
1. Heat the oil in a skillet over medium heat. Add fennel, onion, and ½ tsp. salt and cook for 5 minutes. Stir in thyme and garlic and cook for 30 seconds.
2. Stir in the wine and tomatoes and then bring to a simmer.
3. Pat the hake dry with paper towels and season with salt and pepper. Place the hake into the skillet (skin side down). Spoon some sauce over the top and bring to a simmer.

4. Lower the heat to medium-low, cover, and cook for 10 to 12 minutes, or until the hake flakes apart when prodded with a knife.
5. Serve the hake into individual bowls. Stir parsley into the sauce and season with salt and pepper to taste. Spoon the sauce over the hake and drizzle with extra oil.
6. Serve.

NUTRITION: Calories: 292 Fat: 11.1g Carb: 11g Protein: 33g

# Pan-Roasted Sea Bass

Preparation Time: 5 minutes

Cooking Time: 10 minutes

Servings: 2

INGREDIENTS
- Skinless sea bass fillets – 4 (4 to 6 ounces) 1 to 1 ½ inches thick
- Salt and pepper
- Sugar – ½ tsp.
- Extra-virgin olive oil – 1 tbsp.
- Lemon wedges

DIRECTIONS
1. Place the oven rack in the middle and preheat the oven to 425F. Pat the sea bass dry with paper towels and season with salt and pepper. On one side of each fillet, sprinkle the sugar evenly.
2. In a skillet, heat the oil over medium-high. Place the sea bass  sugared side down in the skillet and cook for 2 minutes, or until browned.
3. Then flip and transfer the skillet to the oven and roast for 7 to 10 minutes, or until the fish registers 140F.
4. Serve with lemon wedges.

NUTRITION: Calories: 225 Fat: 4.3g Carb: 1g Protein: 45.5g

# Lemon Fruit and Nut Bars

Preparation Time: 15 minutes

Cooking Time: 0 minute

Servings: 10

INGREDIENTS
- ½ Cup Raw Almonds
- ¾ Cup Raw Cashews
- 1 Cup Deglet Noor Dates
- 1 Lemon – Juice and Zest

DIRECTIONS:
1. Ground cashews and almonds in a nourishment processor until they are finely cut. Add dates, lemon juice, and lemon pieces. Beat until all ingredients are mixed.
2. Pour blend between two sheets of cling wrap. Utilize your hands to press and frame the blend into a minimized rectangular shape.
3. Fold the saran wrap over it and refrigerate for 2 hours. This will enable it to solidify and make it simpler to cut into bars.
4. Remove from the cooler and cut into 10 bars. Envelop the bars with cling wrap and store them in the ice chest.

NUTRITION: Calories: 333 Carbs: 45g Fat: 16g Protein: 7g

# Cauliflower Fried Rice with Bacon

Preparation Time: 5 minutes

Cooking Time: 10 minutes

Servings: 4

INGREDIENTS:
- 4 slices bacon
- 1 small onion
- 1 head cauliflower
- 1 cup frozen mixed vegetables
- 1 tsp Bragg's Liquid Amino

DIRECTIONS:
1. In a wok or enormous sauté container over medium flame, cook bacon. Add the onions and pan-fried food until translucent.
2. Set heat to high. Add the shredded cauliflower and pan-fried food for 1 moment. Add water and mixed vegetables, mix well, spread the dish and let the cauliflower blend steam for an additional 3 minutes or until tender.
3. Add Bragg's Liquid Amino. Taste and add salt for extra flavoring as wanted.

NUTRITION: Calories: 492 Carbs: 28g Fat: 22g Protein: 38g

# Halloumi Cheese with Butter-Fried Eggplant

Preparation Time: 5 minutes

Cooking Time: 10 minutes

Servings: 2

INGREDIENTS:
- 1 eggplant
- 3 oz. butter
- 10 oz. halloumi cheese
- 10 black olives
- salt and pepper

DIRECTIONS:
1. Cut the eggplant down the middle, longwise, and cut into pieces which are a big portion and an inch thick. Heat up a healthful dab of butter in an enormous pan.
2. Add the cheese on one side of the dish and eggplant on the other. Season eggplant with salt and pepper
3. Fry over medium-high heat for 5-7minutes. Flip the cheese after three minutes, with the aim that it's darker on the 2 sides. Mix the eggplant now. Present with olives.

NUTRITION: Calories: 110 Carbs: 0g Fat: 9g Protein: 7g

# White Lasagna Stuffed Peppers

Preparation Time:  5 minutes

Cooking Time: 1 hour

Servings: 4

INGREDIENTS:
- 2 large sweet peppers
- 1 tsp garlic salt
- 12 oz. ground turkey
- 3/4 cup ricotta cheese
- 1 cup mozzarella

DIRECTIONS:
1. Preheat stove to 400. Put the cut peppers in a heating dish. Sprinkle with 1/4 tsp garlic salt. Gap the ground turkey between the peppers.
2. Sprinkle with another 1/4 tsp garlic salt. Cook for 30 minutes. Partition the ricotta cheese between the peppers. Sprinkle with 1/2 tsp garlic salt. Sprinkle the mozzarella on top.
3. Put the cherry tomatoes in the middle of the peppers, if utilizing. Cook for an extra 30 minutes until the meat is cooked, and the cheese is golden.

NUTRITION: Calories: 297 Carbs: 8g Fat: 18g Protein: 25g

# Boiled Eggs with Butter and Thyme

Preparation Time: 10 minutes

Cooking Time: 6 minutes

Servings: 1

INGREDIENTS:
- 3 large eggs
- 1 tbsp. good quality unsalted butter
- Freshly ground black pepper
- Salt
- 1/4 tsp thyme leaves

DIRECTIONS:
1. Fill a medium pan most of the way with water and heat until boiling. When water is bubbling, tenderly put eggs in water and flip using a large spoon.
2. While your eggs are cooking, place one tsp of margarine in a microwave-safe bowl and microwave until dissolved, for around 20 seconds.
3. In the meantime, take the pan and cautiously spill out the excessive water carefully.
4. Cautiously remove shell from every egg, wash to remove any shell parts, and add in the softened margarine. Add the thyme leaves as well as the salt and pepper for flavor.

NUTRITION: Calories: 160 Carbs: 1g Fat: 12g Protein: 14g

# Fluffy Microwave Scrambled Eggs

Preparation Time: 5 minutes

Cooking Time: 5 minutes

Servings: 2

INGREDIENTS:
- 4 eggs
- 1/4 cup milk
- 1/8 teaspoon salt

DIRECTIONS:
1. Break the eggs into a microwavable bowl. Add milk and salt; blend well. Pop the bowl into the microwave and cook on high for 30 seconds.
2. Remove the bowl, beat eggs well overall, scratching down the sides of the bowl, and place back into the microwave for an additional 30 seconds.
3. Repeat this example, blending like clockwork for up to 2 1/2 minutes. Stop when eggs have the consistency you want.

NUTRITION: Calories: 67 Carbs: 1g Fat: 4g Protein: 6g

# Caesar Salad Deviled Eggs

Preparation Time: 120 minutes

Cooking Time: 10 minutes

Servings: 4

INGREDIENTS:
- 6 large pastured eggs
- 1/3 cup creamy Caesar dressing
- 1/2 cup Parmesan cheese
- Cracked black pepper
- 1 romaine lettuce leaf

DIRECTIONS:
1. In a blending bowl, crush the egg yolks with a fork. Add Caesar dressing, 1/4 cup of the Parmesan cheddar and half of the chopped lettuce, then mix.
2. Utilize a baked good sack to pipe the blend into the egg whites. Top each egg with a little Parmesan cheddar, shredded lettuce and black pepper.

NUTRITION: Calories: 80 Carbs: 1g Fat: 7g Protein: 3g

# Caesar Egg Salad Lettuce Wraps

Preparation Time: 10 minutes

Cooking Time: 10 minutes

Servings: 4

INGREDIENTS:
- 6 large hard-boiled eggs
- 3 tbsp. creamy Caesar and 3 tbsp. mayonnaise
- 1/2 cup Parmesan cheese
- Cracked black pepper
- 4 large romaine lettuce leaves

DIRECTIONS:
1. In a blending bowl, mix eggs, velvety Caesar dressing, mayonnaise, 1/4 cup Parmesan cheddar and black pepper.
2. Spoon blend into a mixture of romaine leaves and top with residual Parmesan cheddar.

NUTRITION: Calories: 270 Carbs: 1g Fat: 20g Protein: 34g

# Sour Cream and Chive Egg Clouds

Preparation Time: 10 minutes

Cooking Time: 6 minutes

Servings: 4

INGREDIENTS:
- 8 large pastured eggs
- 1/4 cup sharp white cheddar cheese
- 1/4 cup sour cream
- 1 tsp garlic powder
- 2 chives and 2 tsp salted butter

DIRECTIONS:
1. Preheat stove to 450º. Line an oven tray with parchment paper. Separate the eggs, emptying the whites into an enormous blending bowl, and the yolks into singular ramekins.
2. Utilizing an electric blender, whip the egg whites until they are fleecy and solid pinnacles have begun to frame.
3. Utilizing an elastic spatula, delicately overlap in cheddar, cream, garlic powder, and half of the chives.
4. Spoon blend into 8 separate hills on the parchment paper. Make a hole in the focal point of each cloud.
5. Heat for 6 minutes or until the mists are golden on top and the yolks are set. Put a modest quantity of margarine over every yolk. Top with chives. Serve and Enjoy

NUTRITION: Calories: 101 Carbs: 18g Fat: 2g
Protein: 2g

# Bacon-Wrapped Avocado Fries

Preparation Time: 10 minutes

Cooking Time: 10 minutes

Servings: 20

INGREDIENTS :
- 20 strips of pre-cooked packaged bacon
- 1 large avocado sliced into thin fry-size pieces

DIRECTIONS:
1. Preheat stove to 425°F. Take one strip of precooked bacon and attempt to tenderly stretch somewhat longer without it breaking.
2. Cautiously fold-over avocado, beginning toward one side and attempting to the opposite end. Repeat with remaining ingredients and put onto an oven tray. Heat for 5-10 minutes and serve.

NUTRITION:  Calories: 231 Carbs: 2g Fat: 19g Protein: 9g

# Couscous and Tomato Salad

Preparation time: 10 minutes

Cooking time:  6 minutes

Servings : 4

INGREDIENTS:
- 1/3 cup couscous
- 1/3 cup chicken stock
- ¼ teaspoon ground black pepper
- ¾ teaspoon ground coriander
- ½ teaspoon salt
- ¼ teaspoon paprika
- ¼ teaspoon turmeric
- 1 tablespoon butter
- 2 oz chickpeas, canned, drained
- 1 cup fresh arugula, chopped
- 2 oz sun-dried tomatoes, chopped
- 1 oz Feta cheese, crumbled
- 1 tablespoon canola oil

DIRECTIONS:
1. Bring the chicken stock to boil. Add couscous, ground black pepper, ground coriander, salt, paprika, and turmeric. Add chickpeas and butter. Stir the mixture well and close the lid.
2. Let the couscous soak the hot chicken stock for 6 minutes. Meanwhile, in the mixing bowl combine together arugula, sun -dried tomatoes, and Feta cheese.
3. Add cooked couscous mixture and canola oil. Mix up the salad well.

NUTRITION: Calories 187 Fat 9g Carbs 21.1g
Protein 6g

# Orange Couscous

Preparation time: 5 minutes

Cooking time: 15 minutes

Servings: 2

INGREDIENTS:
- 1/3 cup couscous
- ¼ cup of water
- 4 tablespoons orange juice
- ¼ orange, chopped
- 1 teaspoon Italian seasonings
- 1/3 teaspoon salt
- ½ teaspoon butter

DIRECTIONS:
1. Pour water and orange juice in the pan. Add orange, Italian seasoning, and salt. Bring the liquid to boil and remove it from the heat.
2. Add butter and couscous. Stir well and close the lid. Leave the couscous rest for 10 minutes.

NUTRITION: Calories 149 Fat 1.9g Carbs 28.5g Protein 4.1g

# Paprika Couscous

Preparation time: 15 minutes
Cooking time : 7.5 hours

Servings: 4

INGREDIENTS:
- 1 cup couscous
- 3 ½ cup chicken stock
- ½ cup mascarpone
- 1 teaspoon salt
- 1 teaspoon ground paprika

DIRECTIONS:
1. Place chicken stock and mascarpone in the pan and bring the liquid to boil. Add salt and ground paprika. Stir gently and simmer for 1 minute.
2. Remove the liquid from the heat and add couscous. Stir well and close the lid. Leave couscous for 10 minutes. Stir the cooked side dish well before serving.

NUTRITION: Calories 227 Fat 4.9g Carbs 35.4g Protein 9.7g

# Chili Corn Mix

Preparation time : 8 minutes

Cooking time: 5 minutes

Servings: 3

INGREDIENTS:
- 1 cup corn kernels
- 1 tablespoon coconut flour
- ½ teaspoon salt
- 3 tablespoons canola oil
- ½ teaspoon ground paprika
- ¾ teaspoon chili pepper
- 1 tablespoon water

DIRECTIONS:
1. In the mixing bowl combine together corn kernels with salt and coconut flour. Add water and mix up the corn with the help of the spoon.
2. Pour canola oil in the skillet and heat it up. Add corn kernels mixture and roast it for 4 minutes. Stir it from time to time.
3. When the corn kernels are crunchy, transfer them in the plate and dry with the help of the paper towel. Add chili pepper and ground paprika. Mix up well.

NUTRITION: Calories 179 Fat 15g Carbs 11.3g Protein 2.1g

# Corn and Tomato Salad

Preparation time : 10 minutes
Cooking time : 0 minutes

Servings: 4

INGREDIENTS:
- ¼ cup Greek yogurt
- 1 cup shoepeg corn, drained
- ½ cup cherry tomatoes halved
- 1 jalapeno pepper, chopped
- 1 tablespoon lemon juice
- 3 tablespoons fresh cilantro, chopped
- 1 tablespoon chives, chopped

DIRECTIONS:
1. In the salad bowl mix up together shoepeg corn, cherry tomatoes, jalapeno pepper, chives, and fresh cilantro. Add lemon juice and Greek yogurt. Mix the salad well. Store it in the fridge up to 1 day.

NUTRITION: Calories 49 Fat 0.7g Carbs 9.4g Protein 2.7g

# Lemon Farro

Preparation time: 10 minutes

Cooking time: 35 minutes

Servings: 2

INGREDIENTS:
- ½ cup farro
- 1 ½ cup chicken stock
- 1 teaspoon salt
- ½ teaspoon ground black pepper
- 2 cups arugula, chopped
- 1 cucumber, chopped
- 1 tablespoon lemon juice
- ½ teaspoon olive oil
- ½ teaspoon Italian seasoning

DIRECTIONS:
1. Mix up together farro, salt, and chicken stock and transfer mixture in the pan. Close the lid and boil it for 35 minutes.
2. Meanwhile, place all remaining ingredients in the salad bowl. Chill the farro to the room temperature and add it in the salad bowl too. Mix up the salad well.

NUTRITION: Calories 92 Fat 2.3 Carbs 15.6 Protein 3.9

# Turmeric Farro and Carrot

Preparation time: 5 minutes

Cooking time: 35 minutes

Servings: 2

INGREDIENTS:
- ½ cup farro
- 1 ½ cup water
- 1 teaspoon salt
- 1 teaspoon chili flakes
- ½ teaspoon paprika
- ½ teaspoon turmeric
- ½ teaspoon ground coriander
- 1 yellow onion, sliced
- 1 tablespoon butter
- 1 carrot, grated

DIRECTIONS:
1. Place farro in the pan. Add water and salt. Close the lid and boil it for 30 minutes. Meanwhile, toss the butter in the skillet.
2. Heat it up and add sliced onion and grated carrot. Fry the vegetables for 10 minutes over the medium heat. Stir them with the help of spatula from time to time.
3. When the farro is cooked, add it in the roasted vegetables and mix up well. Cook stir-fried farro for 5 minutes over the medium-high heat.

NUTRITION: Calories 129 Fat 5.9g Carbs 17.1g Protein 2.8g

# Mushroom Risotto

Preparation time: 10 minutes

Cooking time: 55 minutes

Servings: 4

INGREDIENTS:
- 1 cup farro
- 4 cups chicken stock
- 2 oz Parmesan, shaved
- 1 teaspoon ground thyme
- 1 teaspoon ground black pepper
- ½ teaspoon chili flakes
- ½ teaspoon paprika
- ½ teaspoon ground coriander
- 1 teaspoon dried oregano
- 1 tablespoon butter
- 1 yellow onion, diced
- ½ cup cremini mushrooms, sliced
- ¼ cup heavy cream

DIRECTIONS:
1. Toss butter in the saucepan and heat it up. Add onion and mushrooms. Sauté the vegetables for 10 minutes over the medium heat.
2. Then sprinkle them with ground thyme, ground black pepper, chili flakes, paprika, ground coriander, and dried oregano. Mix up well.
3. After this, add the farro and roast the ingredients for 5 minutes. Stir them from time to time with the help of a spatula.

4. Then add heavy cream, chicken stock, and Parmesan. Mix up well and close the lid. Sauté risotto for 40 minutes over the medium-low heat.

NUTRITION: Calories 164 Fat 9.4g Carbs 13.5g Protein 7.9g

# Cheesy Barley

Preparation time: 10 minutes
Cooking time : 45 minutes

Servings: 8

INGREDIENTS:
- 2 cups of water
- 1 cup barley
- 1 teaspoon salt
- 1 cup Cheddar cheese, shredded
- 1/3 cup Mozzarella cheese, shredded
- 1 cup milk
- 1 tablespoon butter
- 1 tablespoon fresh cilantro, chopped
- 1/3 cup fresh parsley, chopped
- 1 teaspoon ground black pepper
- ½ teaspoon minced garlic
- 2 tablespoons almond flour

DIRECTIONS:
1. Place barley and water in the pan and bring them to boil. Close the lid and cook the barley for 20 minutes.
2. Meanwhile, combine together Cheddar cheese, Mozzarella cheese, milk, fresh cilantro, parsley, ground black pepper, and minced garlic. Mix up the mixture well.
3. Rub the gratin mold with butter generously. Then make the layer of barley inside it. After this, pour the cheese mixture over the barley and flatten it well with the help of the spatula.
4. Sprinkle the top of the gratin with almond flour. Bake the gratin for 25 minutes at

355F. Serve.
NUTRITION: Calories 212 Fat 11g Carbs 14.9g
Protein 6.8g

# Kale and Spinach Mix

Preparation time: 10 minutes

Cooking time: 45 minutes

Servings: 4

INGREDIENTS:
- 1 cup kale, chopped
- ½ cup fresh spinach, chopped
- ¼ cup fresh dill, chopped
- 1 teaspoon salt
- 1 bay leaf
- 6 cups beef broth
- 3 tablespoons chives, chopped
- ¼ cup barley
- 1 teaspoon white pepper
- ¾ teaspoon cayenne pepper
- 1/3 cup mushrooms, chopped
- 1 teaspoon olive oil

DIRECTIONS:
1. Pour beef broth in the pan and bring it to boil. Meanwhile, pour olive oil in the skillet. Add mushrooms and cayenne pepper.
2. Roast the vegetables for 7 minutes. Stir them from time to time. Then transfer the mushrooms in the boiling beef broth. Add barley and boil the sauté for 25 minutes.
3. After this, add fresh dill, fresh spinach, salt, bay leaf, and kale. Add chives and cook sauté for 10 minutes more. Then remove the bay leaf and close the lid.
4. Let the cooked sauté rest for 10-15 minutes before serving. Serve the sauté in

the serving bowls.
NUTRITION: Calories 130 Fat 3.8g Carbs 14.4g
Protein 10.3g

# Cabbage and Mushrooms Mix

Preparation time: 10 minutes

Cooking time: 15 minutes

Servings: 2

INGREDIENTS:
- 1 yellow onion, sliced
- 2 tablespoons olive oil
- 1 tablespoon balsamic vinegar
- ½ pound white mushrooms, sliced
- 1 green cabbage head, shredded
- 4 spring onions, chopped
- Salt and black pepper to the taste

DIRECTIONS:
1. Heat up a pan with the oil over medium heat, add the yellow onion and the spring onions and cook for 5 minutes.
2. Add the rest of the ingredients, cook everything for 10 minutes, divide between plates and serve.

NUTRITION: Calories 199 Fat 4.5g Carbs 5.6g Protein 2.2g

# Lemon Mushroom Rice

Preparation time: 1 0 minutes

Cooking time: 30 minutes

Servings: 4

INGREDIENTS:
- 2 cups chicken stock
- 1 yellow onion, chopped
- ½ pound white mushrooms, sliced
- 2 garlic cloves, minced
- 8 ounces wild rice
- Juice and zest of 1 lemon
- 1 tablespoon chives, chopped
- 6 tablespoons goat cheese, crumbled
- Salt and black pepper to the taste

DIRECTIONS:
1. Heat up a pot with the stock over medium heat, add the rice, onion and the rest of the ingredients except the chives and the cheese, bring to a simmer and cook for 25 minutes.
2. Add the remaining ingredients, cook everything for 5 minutes, divide between plates and serve as a side dish.

NUTRITION: Calories 222 Fat 5.5g Carbs 12.3g Protein 5.6g

# Paprika and Chives Potatoes

Preparation time: 10 minutes
Cooking time: 1 hour and 8 minutes

Servings: 4

INGREDIENTS:
- 4 potatoes, scrubbed and pricked with a fork
- 1 tablespoon olive oil
- 1 celery stalk, chopped
- 2 tomatoes, chopped
- 1 teaspoon sweet paprika
- Salt and black pepper to the taste
- 2 tablespoons chives, chopped

DIRECTIONS:
1. Arrange the potatoes on a baking sheet lined with parchment paper, introduce in the oven and bake at 350 degrees F for 1 hour.
2. Cool the potatoes down, peel and cut them into larger cubes. Heat up a pan with the oil over medium heat, add the celery and the tomatoes and sauté for 2 minutes.
3. Add the potatoes and the rest of the ingredients, toss, cook everything for 6 minutes, divide the mix between plates and serve as a side dish.

NUTRITION: Calories 233 Fat 8.7g Carbs 14.4g Protein 6.4g

# Bulgur, Kale and Cheese Mix

Preparation time: 10 minutes

Cooking time: 10 minutes

Servings: 6

INGREDIENTS:
- 4 ounces bulgur
- 4 ounces kale, chopped
- 1 tablespoon mint, chopped
- 3 spring onions, chopped
- 1 cucumber, chopped
- A pinch of allspice, ground
- 2 tablespoons olive oil
- Zest and juice of ½ lemon
- 4 ounces feta cheese, crumbled

DIRECTIONS:
1. Put bulgur in a bowl, cover with hot water, aside for 10 minutes and fluff with a fork. Heat up a pan with the oil over medium heat, add the onions and the allspice and cook for 3 minutes.
2. Add the bulgur and the rest of the ingredients, cook everything for 5-6 minutes more, divide between plates and serve.

NUTRITION: Calories 200 Fat 6.7g Carbs 15.4g Protein 4.5g

# Spicy Green Beans Mix

Preparation time: 5 minutes

Cooking time: 15 minutes

Servings: 4

INGREDIENTS:
- 4 teaspoons olive oil
- 1 garlic clove, minced
- ½ teaspoon hot paprika
- ¾ cup veggie stock
- 1 yellow onion, sliced
- 1-pound green beans, trimmed and halved
- ½ cup goat cheese, shredded
- 2 teaspoon balsamic vinegar

DIRECTIONS:
1. Heat up a pan with the oil over medium heat, add the garlic, stir and cook for 1 minute.
2. Add the green beans and the rest of the ingredients, toss, cook everything for 15 minutes more, divide between plates and serve as a side dish.

NUTRITION: Calories 188 Fat 4g Carbs 12.4g Protein 4.4g

# Beans and Rice

Preparation time: 10 minutes

Cooking time: 55 minutes

Servings: 6

INGREDIENTS:
- 1 tablespoon olive oil
- 1 yellow onion, chopped
- 2 celery stalks, chopped
- 2 garlic cloves, minced
- 2 cups brown rice
- 1 and ½ cup canned black beans, rinsed and drained
- 4 cups water
- Salt and black pepper to the taste

DIRECTIONS:
1. Heat up a pan with the oil over medium heat, add the celery, garlic and the onion, stir and cook for 10 minutes.
2. Add the rest of the ingredients, stir, bring to a simmer and cook over medium heat for 45 minutes. Divide between plates and serve.

NUTRITION: Calories 224 Fat 8.4g Carbs 15.3g Protein 6.2g

# Tomato and Millet Mix

Preparation time: 10 minutes

Cooking time: 20 minutes

Servings: 6

INGREDIENTS:
- 3 tablespoons olive oil
- 1 cup millet
- 2 spring onions, chopped
- 2 tomatoes, chopped
- ½ cup cilantro, chopped
- 1 teaspoon chili paste
- 6 cups cold water
- ½ cup lemon juice
- Salt and black pepper to the taste

DIRECTIONS:
1. Heat up a pan with the oil over medium heat, add the millet, stir and cook for 4 minutes. Add the water, salt and pepper, stir, bring to a simmer over medium heat cook for 15 minutes.
2. Add the rest of the ingredients, toss, divide the mix between plates and serve as a side dish.

NUTRITION: Calories 222 Fat 10.2g Carbs 14.5g Protein 2.4g

# Quinoa and Greens Salad

Preparation time: 10 minutes
Cooking time : 0 minutes

Servings: 4

INGREDIENTS:
- 1 cup quinoa, cooked
- 1 medium bunch collard greens, chopped
- 4 tablespoons walnuts, chopped
- 2 tablespoons balsamic vinegar
- 4 tablespoons tahini paste
- 4 tablespoons cold water
- A pinch of salt and black pepper
- 1 tablespoon olive oil

DIRECTIONS:
1. In a bowl, mix the tahini with the water and vinegar and whisk.
2. In a bowl, mix the quinoa with the rest of the ingredients and the tahini dressing, toss, divide the mix between plates and serve as a side dish.

NUTRITION: Calories 175 Fat 3g Carbs 5g Protein 3g

# Veggies and Avocado Dressing

Preparation time: 10 minutes

Cooking time: 0 minutes

Servings: 4

INGREDIENTS:
- 3 tablespoons pepitas, roasted
- 3 cups water
- 2 tablespoons cilantro, chopped
- 4 tablespoons parsley, chopped
- 1 and ½ cups corn
- 1 cup radish, sliced
- 2 avocados, peeled, pitted and chopped
- 2 mangos, peeled and chopped
- 3 tablespoons olive oil
- 4 tablespoons Greek yogurt
- 1 teaspoon balsamic vinegar
- 2 tablespoons lime juice
- Salt and black pepper to the taste

DIRECTIONS:
1. In your blender, mix the olive oil with avocados, salt, pepper, lime juice, the yogurt and the vinegar and pulse.
2. In a bowl, mix the pepitas with the cilantro, parsley and the rest of the ingredients, and toss. Add the avocado dressing, toss, divide the mix between plates and serve as a side dish.

NUTRITION: Calories 403 Fat 30.5g Carbs 23.5g Protein 3.5g

# Dill Beets Salad

Preparation time: 10 minutes
Cooking time : 0 minutes

Servings: 6

INGREDIENTS:
- 2 pounds beets, cooked, peeled and cubed
- 2 tablespoons olive oil
- 1 tablespoon lemon juice
- 2 tablespoons balsamic vinegar
- 1 cup feta cheese, crumbled
- 3 small garlic cloves, minced
- 4 green onions, chopped
- 5 tablespoons parsley, chopped
- Salt and black pepper to the taste

DIRECTIONS:
1. In a bowl, mix the beets with the oil, lemon juice and the rest of the ingredients, toss and serve as a side dish.

NUTRITION: Calories 268 Fat 15.5g Carbs 25.7g Protein 9.6g

# Brussels Sprouts Hash

Preparation time: 10 minutes

Cooking time: 20 minutes

Servings: 4

INGREDIENTS:
- 3 tablespoons extra-virgin olive oil
- 1 onion, finely chopped
- 1 pound Brussels sprouts, bottoms trimmed off, shredded (see tip)
- ½ teaspoon caraway seeds
- ½ teaspoon sea salt
- 1/8 teaspoon freshly ground black pepper
- ¼ cup red wine vinegar
- 1 tablespoon Dijon mustard
- 1 tablespoon honey
- 3 garlic cloves, minced

DIRECTIONS:
2. In a large skillet over medium-high heat, heat the olive oil until it shimmers. Add the onion, Brussels sprouts, caraway seeds, sea salt, and pepper.
3. Cook for 7 to 10 minutes, stirring occasionally, until the Brussels sprouts begin to brown. While the Brussels sprouts cook, whisk the vinegar, mustard, and honey in a small bowl and set aside.
4. Add the garlic to the skillet and cook for 30 seconds, stirring constantly. Add the vinegar mixture to the skillet. Cook for about 5 minutes, stirring, until the liquid reduces by half.

NUTRITION: Calories: 176 Protein: 11g
Carbohydrates: 19g Fat: 11g

# Roasted Asparagus with Lemon and Pine Nuts

Preparation time: 5 minutes

Cooking time: 20 minutes

Servings: 4

INGREDIENTS:
- 1 pound asparagus, trimmed
- 2 tablespoons extra-virgin olive oil
- Juice of 1 lemon
- Zest of 1 lemon
- ¼ cup pine nuts
- ½ teaspoon sea salt
- 1/8 teaspoon freshly ground black pepper

DIRECTIONS:
1. Preheat the oven to 425°F. In a large bowl, toss the asparagus with the olive oil, lemon juice and zest, pine nuts, sea salt, and pepper.
2. Spread in a roasting pan in an even layer. Roast for about 20 minutes until the asparagus is browned.

NUTRITION: Calories: 144 Protein: 4g
Carbohydrates: 6g Fat: 13g

# Citrus Sautéed Spinach

Preparation time: 5 minutes

Cooking time: 5 minutes

Servings: 4

INGREDIENTS:
1. 2 tablespoons extra-virgin olive oil
2. 4 cups fresh baby spinach
3. 1 teaspoon orange zest
4. ¼ cup freshly squeezed orange juice
5. ½ teaspoon sea salt
6. 1/8 teaspoon freshly ground black pepper

DIRECTIONS:
1. In a large skillet over medium-high heat, heat the olive oil until it shimmers. Add the spinach and orange zest. Cook for about 3 minutes, stirring occasionally, until the spinach wilts.
2. Stir in the orange juice, sea salt, and pepper. Cook for 2 minutes more, stirring occasionally. Serve hot.

NUTRITION: Calories: 74 Protein: 7g
Carbohydrates: 3g Fat: 7g

# Mashed Cauliflower

Preparation time: 10 minutes

Cooking time: 15 minutes

Servings: 4

INGREDIENTS:
- 4 cups cauliflower florets
- ¼ cup skim milk
- ¼ cup (2 ounces) grated Parmesan cheese
- 2 tablespoons butter
- 2 tablespoons extra-virgin olive oil
- ½ teaspoon sea salt
- 1/8 teaspoon freshly ground black pepper

DIRECTIONS:
1. In a large pot over medium-high, cover the cauliflower with water and bring it to a boil. Reduce the heat to medium-low, cover, and simmer for about 10 minutes until the cauliflower is soft.
2. Drain the cauliflower and return it to the pot. Add the milk, cheese, butter, olive oil, sea salt, and pepper. Using a potato masher, mash until smooth.

NUTRITION: Calories: 187 Protein: 7g
Carbohydrates: 7g Fat: 16g

# Broccoli with Ginger and Garlic

Preparation time: 10 minutes

Cooking time: 11 minutes

Servings: 4

INGREDIENTS:
- 2 tablespoons extra-virgin olive oil
- 2 cups broccoli florets
- 1 tablespoon grated fresh ginger
- ½ teaspoon sea salt
- 1/8 teaspoon freshly ground black pepper
- 3 garlic cloves, minced

DIRECTIONS:
1. In a large skillet over medium-high heat, heat the olive oil until it shimmers. Add the broccoli, ginger, sea salt, and pepper.
2. Cook for about 10 minutes, stirring occasionally, until the broccoli is soft and starts to brown. Add the garlic and cook for 30 seconds, stirring constantly. Remove from the heat and serve.

NUTRITION: Calories: 80 Protein: 1g
Carbohydrates: 4g Fat: 0g

# Balsamic Roasted Carrots

Preparation time: 10 minutes

Cooking time: 30 minutes

Servings: 4

INGREDIENTS:
- 1½ pounds carrots, quartered lengthwise
- 2 tablespoons extra-virgin olive oil
- ¼ teaspoon sea salt
- 1/8 teaspoon freshly ground black pepper
- 3 tablespoons balsamic vinegar

DIRECTIONS:
1. Preheat the oven to 425°F. In a large bowl, toss the carrots with the olive oil, sea salt, and pepper. Place in a single layer in a roasting pan or on a rimmed baking sheet.
2. Roast for 20 to 30 minutes until the carrots are caramelized. Toss with the vinegar and serve.

NUTRITION: Calories: 132 Protein: 1g
Carbohydrates: 17g Fat: 7g

# Parmesan Zucchini Sticks

Preparation time: 10 minutes

Cooking time: 20 minutes

Servings: 4

INGREDIENT s:
- 4 zucchinis, quartered lengthwise
- 2 tablespoons extra-virgin olive oil
- ½ cup (4 ounces) grated Parmesan cheese
- 1 tablespoon Italian seasoning
- ½ teaspoon sea salt
- ¼ teaspoon garlic powder
- 1/8 teaspoon freshly ground black pepper

DIRECTIONS:
1. Preheat the oven to 350°F. In a large bowl, toss the zucchini with the olive oil. In a small bowl, whisk the cheese, Italian seasoning, sea salt, garlic powder, and pepper. Toss with the zucchini.
2. Place the zucchini in a single layer on a rimmed baking sheet. Bake for 15 to 20 minutes until the zucchini is soft.
3. Set the oven to broil, and broil for 1 to 2 minutes until the cheese-herb coating crisps, watching carefully so it doesn't burn.

NUTRITION: Calories: 194 Protein: 12g
Carbohydrates: 8g  Fat: 14g

# Basmati Rice

Preparation time: 7 minutes

Cooking time: 20 minutes

Servings: 4

INGREDIENTS:
- 1 cup basmati rice
- 2 tablespoons olive oil
- 1 teaspoon salt
- 2 ½ cup chicken stock

DIRECTIONS:
1. Pour olive oil in the pan and heat it up. Add basmati rice and roast it for 3 minutes. Stir it from time to time. Then add salt and chicken stock.
2. Mix up the ingredients until homogenous. Close the lid and boil rice for 15 minutes or until it soaks all the liquid.

NUTRITION: Calories 235 Fat 7.7g Carbs 37.4g Protein 3.7g

# Spiced Buckwheat

Preparation time: 10 minutes

Cooking time: 25 minutes

Servings: 4

INGREDIENTS:
- ½ teaspoon ground cardamom
- ¾ teaspoon ground cinnamon
- ¾ teaspoon ground ginger
- 1 teaspoon salt
- 2 tablespoons butter
- 1 tablespoon olive oil
- 1 ½ cup buckwheat
- 3 cups beef broth

DIRECTIONS:
1. Place olive oil in the pan and heat it up. Add buckwheat and butter. Roast the buckwheat for 5 minutes over the medium heat. Stir it from time to time.
2. Then add ground cardamom, ground cinnamon, salt, and ginger. Mix up the buckwheat. Add beef broth, mix up, and cook buckwheat for 20 minutes over the low heat. Serve.

NUTRITION: Calories 331 Fat 12.5g Carbs 47g Protein 12.2g

# Coconut Bulgur

Preparation time: 7 minutes

Cooking time: 20 minutes

Servings: 2

INGREDIENTS:
- ½ cup bulgur
- 1 teaspoon tomato paste
- ½ white onion, diced
- 2 tablespoons coconut oil
- 1 ½ cup chicken stock

DIRECTIONS:
1. Toss coconut oil in the pan and melt it. Add diced onion and roast it until light brown. Then add bulgur and stir well. Cook bulgur in coconut oil for 3 minutes.
2. Then add tomato paste and mix up bulgur until homogenous. Add chicken stock. Close the lid and cook bulgur for 15 minutes over the medium heat. The cooked bulgur should soak all liquid.

NUTRITION: Calories 257 Fat 14.5g Carbs 30.2g Protein 5.2g

# Cardamom Couscous

Preparation time: 10 minutes

Cooking time: 10 minutes

Servings: 4

INGREDIENTS:
- 1 cup yellow couscous
- ½ teaspoon ground cardamom
- 1 cup chicken stock
- 1 tablespoon butter
- 1 teaspoon salt
- ½ teaspoon red pepper

DIRECTIONS:
1. Toss butter in the pan and melt it. Add couscous and roast it for 1 minute over the high heat. Then add ground cardamom, salt, and red pepper. Stir it well.
2. Add chicken stock and bring the mixture to boil. Simmer couscous for 5 minutes with the closed lid.

NUTRITION: Calories 196 Fat 3.4g Carbs 35g Protein 5.9g

# Parmesan Polenta

Preparation time: 8 minutes

Cooking time: 45 minutes

Servings: 4

INGREDIENTS:
- 1 cup polenta
- 1 ½ cup water
- 2 cups chicken stock
- ½ cup cream
- 1/3 cup Parmesan, grated

DIRECTIONS:
1. Put polenta in the pot. Add water, chicken stock, cream, and Parmesan. Mix up polenta well. Then preheat oven to 355F.
2. Cook polenta in the oven for 45 minutes. Mix up the cooked meal with the help of the spoon carefully before serving.

NUTRITION: Calories 208 Fat 5.3g Carbs 32.2g Protein 8g

# Buttery Millet

Preparation time: 10 minutes

Cooking time: 15 minutes

Servings: 3

INGREDIENTS:
- ¼ cup mushrooms, sliced
- ¾ cup onion, diced
- 1 tablespoon olive oil
- 1 teaspoon salt
- 3 tablespoons milk
- ½ cup millet
- 1 cup of water
- 1 teaspoon butter

DIRECTIONS:
1. Pour olive oil in the skillet and add the onion. Add mushrooms and roast the vegetables for 10 minutes over the medium heat. Stir them from time to time.
2. Meanwhile, pour water in the pan. Add millet and salt. Cook the millet with the closed lid for 15 minutes over the medium heat.
3. Then add the cooked mushroom mixture in the millet. Add milk and butter. Mix up the millet well.

NUTRITION: Calories 198 Fat 7.7g Carbs 27.9g Protein 4.7g

# Cayenne Barley

Preparation time: 7 minutes

Cooking time: 42 minutes

Servings: 5

INGREDIENTS:
- 1 cup barley
- 3 cups chicken stock
- ½ teaspoon cayenne pepper
- 1 teaspoon salt
- ½ teaspoon chili pepper
- ½ teaspoon ground black pepper
- 1 teaspoon butter
- 1 teaspoon olive oil

DIRECTIONS:
1. Place barley and olive oil in the pan. Roast barley on high heat for 1 minute. Stir it well. Then add salt, chili pepper, ground black pepper, cayenne pepper, and butter.
2. Add chicken stock. Close the lid and cook barley for 40 minutes over the medium-low heat.

NUTRITION: Calories 152 Fat 2.9g Carbs 27.8g Protein 5.1g

# Dill Farro

Preparation time : 8 minutes

Cooking time: 40 minutes

Servings:  4

INGREDIENTS:
- 1 cup farro
- 3 cups beef broth
- 1 teaspoon salt
- 1 tablespoon almond butter
- 1 tablespoon dried dill

DIRECTIONS:
1. Place farro in the pan. Add beef broth, dried dill, and salt. Close the lid and bring the mixture to boil. Then boil it for 35 minutes over the medium-low heat.
2. When the time is over, open the lid and add almond butter. Mix up the cooked farro well.

NUTRITION: Calories 95 Fat 3.3g Carbs 10.1g Protein 6.4g

# Wheatberry and Walnuts Salad

Preparation time: 10 minutes

Cooking time: 50 minutes

Servings: 2

INGREDIENTS:
- ¼ cup of wheat berries
- 1 cup of water
- 1 teaspoon salt
- 2 tablespoons walnuts, chopped
- 1 tablespoon chives, chopped
- ¼ cup fresh parsley, chopped
- 2 oz pomegranate seeds
- 1 tablespoon canola oil
- 1 teaspoon chili flakes

DIRECTIONS:
1. Place wheat berries and water in the pan. Add salt and simmer the ingredients for 50 minutes over the medium heat.
2. Meanwhile, mix up together walnuts, chives, parsley, pomegranate seeds, and chili flakes. When the wheatberry is cooked, transfer it in the walnut mixture. Add canola oil and mix up the salad well.

NUTRITION: Calories 160 Fat 11.8g Carbs 12g Protein 3.4g

# Curry Rice

Preparation time: 10 minutes
Cooking time: 1 hour 15 minutes

Servings : 5

INGREDIENTS:
- 1 tablespoon curry paste
- ¼ cup milk
- 1 cup wheatberries
- ½ cup of rice
- 1 teaspoon salt
- 4 tablespoons olive oil
- 6 cups chicken stock

DIRECTIONS:
1. Place wheatberries and chicken stock in the pan. Close the lid and cook the mixture for 1 hour over the medium heat. Then add rice, olive oil, and salt. Stir well.
2. Mix up together milk and curry paste. Add the curry liquid in the rice-wheatberry mixture and stir well. Boil the meal for 15 minutes with the closed lid. When the rice is cooked, all the meal is cooked.

NUTRITION: Calories 232 Fat 15g Carbs 23.5g
Protein 3.9g

MAIN RECIPES: MEAT

## 277. Grilled Chicken Breasts

Preparation Time: 10 minutes
Cooking Time : 15 minutes

Servings: 2

INGREDIENTS:
- Boneless skinless chicken breast, 4.
- Lemon juice, 3 tbsp.
- Olive oil, 3 tbsp.
- Chopped fresh parsley, 3 tbsp.
- Minced garlic cloves, 3.
- Paprika, 1 tsp.
- Dried oregano, ½ tsp.
- Salt and pepper, to taste.

DIRECTIONS:
1. In a large Ziploc bag, mix well oregano, paprika, garlic, parsley, olive oil, and lemon juice.
2. Pierce chicken with a knife several times and sprinkle with salt and pepper.
3. Add chicken to bag and marinate 20 minutes or up to two days in the fridge.
4. Remove chicken from bag and grill for 5 minutes per side in a 350 0 F preheated grill.
5. When cooked, transfer to a plate for 5 minutes before slicing.
6. Serve and enjoy with a side of rice or salad

NUTRITION: Calories: 238, Protein: 24 g, Carbohydrates: 2 g, Fats: 19 g

# Buttery Garlic Chicken

Preparation Time: 5 minutes
Cooking Time : 40 minutes

Servings: 2

INGREDIENTS:
- 2 tablespoons ghee, melted
- 2 boneless skinless chicken breasts
- tablespoon dried Italian seasoning
- 4 tablespoons butter
- ¼ cup grated Parmesan cheese

DIRECTIONS:
1. Preheat the oven to 375°F. Select a baking dish that fit both chicken breasts and coat it with the ghee.
2. Pat dries the chicken breasts. Season with pink Himalayan salt, pepper, and Italian seasoning. Place the chicken in the baking dish.
3. In a medium skillet over medium heat, melt the butter. Sauté minced garlic, for about 5 minutes.
4. Remove the butter-garlic mixture from the heat, and pour it over the chicken breasts.
5. Roast in the oven for 30 to 35 minutes. Sprinkle some of the Parmesan cheese on top of each chicken breast. Let the chicken rest in the baking dish for 5 minutes.
6. Divide the chicken between two plates, spoon the butter sauce over the chicken, and serve.

NUTRITION: 642 Calories 45g Fat 57g Protein

# Creamy Chicken-Spinach Skillet

Preparation Time: 10 minutes

Cooking Time: 17 minutes

Servings: 2

INGREDIENTS:
- Boneless skinless chicken breast, 1 lb.
- Medium diced onion, 1.
- Diced roasted red peppers, 12 oz.
- Chicken stock, 2 ½ cups.
- Baby spinach leaves, 2 cups.
- Cooked pasta, 2 cups.
- Butter, 2 tbsp.
- Minced garlic cloves, 4.
- Cream cheese, 7 oz.
- Salt and pepper, to taste.

DIRECTIONS:
1. Place a saucepan on medium high heat for 2 minutes. Add butter and melt for a minute, swirling to coat the pan.
2. Add chicken to a pan, season with pepper and salt to taste. Cook chicken on high heat for 3 minutes per side.
3. Lower heat to medium and stir in onions, red peppers, and garlic. Sauté for 5 minutes and deglaze pot with a little bit of stock.
4. Whisk in chicken stock and cream cheese. Cook and mix until thoroughly combined.
5. Stir in spinach and adjust seasoning to taste. Cook for 2 minutes or until spinach is

wilted.

6. Serve and enjoy.

NUTRITION: Calories: 484, Protein: 36 g, Carbohydrates: 33 g, Fats: 22 g

# Slow Cooker Mediterranean Beef Roast

Preparation Time : 10 minutes
Cooking Time: 10 hours and 10 minutes

Servings: 2

INGREDIENTS:
- 3 pounds Chuck roast, boneless
- 2 teaspoons Rosemary
- ½ cup Tomatoes, sun-dried and chopped
- 10 cloves Grated garlic
- ½ cup Beef stock
- 2 tablespoons Balsamic vinegar
- ¼ cup Chopped Italian parsley, fresh
- ¼ cup Chopped olives
- 1 teaspoon Lemon zest
- ¼ cup Cheese grits

DIRECTIONS:
1. In the slow cooker, put garlic, sun dried tomatoes, and the beef roast. Add beef stock and Rosemary. Close the cooker and slow cook for 10 hours.
2. After cooking is over, remove the beef, and shred the meet. Discard the fat. Add back the shredded meat to the slow cooker and simmer for 10 minutes.
3. In a small bowl combine lemon zest, parsley, and olives. Cool the mixture until you are ready to serve. Garnish using the refrigerated mix.
4. Serve it over pasta or egg noodles. Top it with cheese grits.

NUTRITION: 314 Calories 19g Fat 1g Carbohydrate 32g Protein 778mg Sodium

# Slow Cooker Mediterranean Beef with Artichokes

Preparation Time : 3 hours and 20 minutes
Cooking Time: 7 hours and 8 minutes

Servings: 2

INGREDIENTS:
- 2 pounds Beef for stew
- 14 ounces Artichoke hearts
- 1 tablespoon Grape seed oil
- 1 Diced onion
- 32 ounces Beef broth
- 4 cloves Garlic, grated
- 14½ ounces Tinned tomatoes, diced
- 15 ounces Tomato sauce
- 1 teaspoon Dried oregano
- ½ cup Pitted, chopped olives
- 1 teaspoon Dried parsley
- 1 teaspoon Dried oregano
- ½ teaspoon Ground cumin
- 1 teaspoon Dried basil
- 1 Bay leaf
- ½ teaspoon Salt

DIRECTIONS :
1. In a large non-stick skillet pour some oil and bring to medium-high heat. Roast the beef until it turns brown on both the sides. Transfer the beef into a slow cooker.

NUTRITION:  314 Calories 19g Fat 1g Carbohydrate 32g Protein 778mg Sodium

# Slow Cooker Meatloaf

Preparation Time: 10 minutes
Cooking Time: 6 hours and 10 minutes

Servings: 2

INGREDIENTS:
- 2 pounds Ground bison
- 1 Grated zucchini
- 2 large Eggs
- Olive oil cooking spray as required
- 1 Zucchini, shredded
- ½ cup Parsley, fresh, finely chopped
- ½ cup Parmesan cheese, shredded
- 3 tablespoons Balsamic vinegar
- 4 Garlic cloves, grated
- 2 tablespoons Onion minced
- 1 tablespoon Dried oregano
- ½ teaspoon Ground black pepper
- ½ teaspoon Kosher salt
- For the topping:
- ¼ cup Shredded Mozzarella cheese
- ¼ cup Ketchup without sugar
- ¼ cup Freshly chopped parsley

DIRECTIONS:
1. Stripe line the inside of a six-quart slow cooker with aluminum foil. Spray non-stick cooking oil over it.
2. In a large bowl combine ground bison or extra lean ground sirloin, zucchini, eggs, parsley, balsamic vinegar, garlic, dried oregano, sea or kosher salt, minced dry onion, and ground black pepper.

3. Situate this mixture into the slow cooker and form an oblong shaped loaf. Cover the cooker, set on a low heat and cook for 6 hours. After cooking, open the cooker and spread ketchup all over the meatloaf.
4. Now, place the cheese above the ketchup as a new layer and close the slow cooker. Let the meatloaf sit on these two layers for about 10 minutes or until the cheese starts to melt. Garnish with fresh parsley, and shredded Mozzarella cheese.

NUTRITION: 320 Calories 2g Fat 4g Carbohydrates 26g Protein 681mg Sodium

# Slow Cooker Mediterranean Beef Hoagies

Preparation Time : 10 minutes

Cooking Time: 13 hours

Servings: 2

INGREDIENTS:
- 3 pounds Beef top round roast fatless
- ½ teaspoon Onion powder
- ½ teaspoon Black pepper
- 3 cups Low sodium beef broth
- 4 teaspoons Salad dressing mix
- 1 Bay leaf
- 1 tablespoon Garlic, minced
- 2 Red bell peppers, thin strips cut
- 16 ounces Pepperoncino
- 8 slices Sargento Provolone, thin
- 2 ounces Gluten-free bread
- ½ teaspoon salt
- For seasoning:
- 1½ tablespoon Onion powder
- 1½ tablespoon Garlic powder
- 2 tablespoon Dried parsley
- 1 tablespoon stevia
- ½ teaspoon Dried thyme
- 1 tablespoon Dried oregano
- 2 tablespoons Black pepper
- 1 tablespoon Salt
- 6 Cheese slices

DIRECTIONS:

1. Dry the roast with a paper towel. Combine black pepper, onion  powder and salt in a small bowl and rub the mixture over the roast.
2. Place the seasoned roast into a slow cooker.
3. Add broth, salad dressing mix, bay leaf, and garlic to the slow cooker. Combine it gently. Close and set to low cooking for 12 hours. After cooking, remove the bay leaf.
4. Take out the cooked beef and shred the beef meet. Put back the shredded beef and add bell peppers and. Add bell peppers and pepperoncino into the slow cooker.
5. Cover the cooker and low cook for 1 hour. Before serving, top each of the bread with 3 ounces of the meat mixture. Top it with a cheese slice. The liquid gravy can be used as a dip.

NUTRITION: 442 Calories 11.5g Fat 37g Carbohydrates 49g Protein 735mg Sodium

# Beef & Bulgur Meatballs

Preparation Time: 20 minutes

Cooking Time: 28 minutes

Servings: 2

INGREDIENTS:
- ¾ cup uncooked bulgur
- 1-pound ground beef
- ¼ cup shallots, minced
- ¼ cup fresh parsley, minced
- ½ teaspoon ground allspice
- ½ teaspoon ground cumin
- ½ teaspoon ground cinnamon
- ¼ teaspoon red pepper flakes, crushed
- Salt, as required
- 1 tablespoon olive oil

DIRECTIONS:
1. In a large bowl of the cold water, soak the bulgur for about 30 minutes. Drain the bulgur well and then, squeeze with your hands to remove the excess water.
2. In a food processor, add the bulgur, beef, shallot, parsley, spices, salt, and pulse until a smooth mixture is formed.
3. Situate the mixture into a bowl and refrigerate, covered for about 30 minutes. Remove from the refrigerator and make equal sized balls from the beef mixture.
4. In a large nonstick skillet, heat the oil over medium-high heat and cook the meatballs in 2 batches for about 13-14 minutes, flipping frequently. Serve warm.

NUTRITION: 228 Calories 7.4g Fat 0.1g
Carbohydrates 3.5g Protein 766mg Sodium

# Tasty Beef and Broccoli

Preparation Time: 10 minutes

Cooking Time: 15 minutes

Servings: 2

INGREDIENTS:
- 1 and ½ lbs. flanks steak
- 1 tbsp. olive oil
- 1 tbsp. tamari sauce
- 1 cup beef stock
- 1-pound broccoli, florets separated

DIRECTIONS:
1. Combine steak strips with oil and tamari, toss and set aside for 10 minutes. Select your instant pot on sauté mode, place beef strips and brown them for 4 minutes on each side.
2. Stir in stock, cover the pot again and cook on high for 8 minutes. Stir in broccoli, cover and cook on high for 4 minutes more.
3. Portion everything between plates and serve. Enjoy!

NUTRITION: 312 Calories 5g Fat 20g Carbohydrates 4g Protein 694mg Sodium

# Soy Sauce Beef Roast

Preparation Time: 8 minutes

Cooking Time: 35 minutes

Servings: 2

INGREDIENTS:
- ½ teaspoon beef bouillon
- 1 ½ teaspoon rosemary
- ½ teaspoon minced garlic
- 2 pounds roast beef
- 1/3 cup soy sauce

DIRECTIONS:
1. Combine the soy sauce, bouillon, rosemary, and garlic together in a mixing bowl.
2. Turn on your instant pot. Place the roast, and pour enough water to cover the roast; gently stir to mix well. Seal it tight.
3. Click "MEAT/STEW" Cooking function; set pressure level to "HIGH" and set the Cooking time to 35 minutes. Let the pressure to build to cook the ingredients. Once done, click "CANCEL" setting then click "NPR" Cooking function to release the pressure naturally.
4. Gradually open the lid, and shred the meat. Mix in the shredded meat back in the potting mix and stir well. Transfer in serving containers. Serve warm.

NUTRITION: 423 Calories 14g Fat 12g Carbohydrates 21g Protein 884mg Sodium

# Mediterranean Grilled Pork Chops

Preparation time: 1 day & 15 minutes

Cooking time: 20 minutes

Servings: 6

INGREDIENTS:
- 2 pork chops
- ¼ cup olive oil
- 2 yellow onions, sliced
- 2 garlic cloves, minced
- 2 teaspoons mustard
- 1 teaspoon sweet paprika
- Salt and black pepper to taste
- ½ teaspoon oregano, dried
- ½ teaspoon thyme, dried
- A pinch of cayenne pepper

DIRECTIONS:
1. In a small bowl, mix oil with garlic, mustard, paprika, black pepper, oregano, thyme and cayenne and whisk well.
2. In a bowl, combine onions with meat and mustard mix, toss to coat, cover and keep in the fridge for 1 day.
3. Place meat on preheated grill pan over medium high heat, season with salt and cook for 10 minutes on each side.
4. Meanwhile, heat a pan over medium heat, add marinated onions, stir and sauté for 4 minutes. Divide pork chops on plates, add sautéed onions on top and serve.

NUTRITION: Calories 234 Fat 3g Carbs 21g Protein 23g

# Simple Pork Stir Fry

Preparation time: 10 minutes

Cooking time: 15 minutes

Servings: 4

INGREDIENTS:
- 4 ounces bacon, chopped
- 4 ounces snow peas
- 2 tablespoons butter
- 1-pound pork loin, cut into thin strips
- 2 cups mushrooms, sliced
- ¾ cup white wine
- ½ cup yellow onion, chopped
- 3 tablespoons sour cream
- Salt and white pepper to taste

DIRECTIONS:
1. Put snow peas in a saucepan, add water to cover, add a pinch of salt, bring to a boil over medium heat, cook until they are soft, drain and leave aside.
2. Heat a pan over medium high heat, add bacon, cook for a few minutes, drain grease, transfer to a bowl and leave aside.
3. Heat a pan with 1 tablespoon butter over medium heat, add pork strips, salt and pepper to taste, brown for a few minutes and transfer to a plate as well.
4. Return pan to medium heat, add remaining butter and melt it. Add onions and mushrooms, stir and cook for 4 minutes.
5. Add wine, and simmer until it's reduced. Add cream, peas, pork, salt and pepper to taste, stir, heat up, divide between plates,

top with bacon and serve.
NUTRITION: Calories 343 Fat 31g Carbs 21g Protein 23g

# Pork and Lentil Soup

Preparation time: 10 minutes

Cooking time: 1 hour

Servings: 6

INGREDIENTS:
- 1 small yellow onion, chopped
- 1 tablespoon olive oil
- 1 and ½ teaspoons basil, chopped
- 1 and ½ teaspoons ginger, grated
- 3 garlic cloves, chopped
- Salt and black pepper to taste
- ½ teaspoon cumin, ground
- 1 carrot, chopped
- 1-pound pork chops, bone-in 3 ounces brown lentils, rinsed
- 3 cups chicken stock
- 2 tablespoons tomato paste
- 2 tablespoons lime juice
- 1 teaspoon red chili flakes, crushed

DIRECTIONS:
1. Heat a saucepan with the oil over medium heat, add garlic, onion, basil, ginger, salt, pepper and cumin, stir well and cook for 6 minutes.
2. Add carrots, stir and cook 5 more minutes. Add pork and brown for a few minutes. Add lentils, tomato paste and stock, stir, bring to a boil, cover pan and simmer for 50 minutes.
3. Transfer pork to a plate, discard bones, shred it and return to pan. Add chili flakes

and lime juice, stir, ladle into bowls and serve.

NUTRITION: Calories 343 Fat 31g Carbs 21g Protein 23g

# Simple Braised Pork

Preparation time: 40 minutes

Cooking time:  1 hour

Servings: 4

INGREDIENTS:
- 2 pounds pork loin roast, boneless and cubed
- 5 tablespoons butter
- Salt and black pepper to taste
- 2 cups chicken stock
- ½ cup dry white wine
- 2 garlic cloves, minced
- 1 teaspoon thyme, chopped
- 1 thyme spring
- 1 bay leaf
- ½ yellow onion, chopped
- 2 tablespoons white flour
- ¾ pound pearl onions
- ½ pound red grapes

DIRECTIONS:
1. Heat a pan with 2 tablespoons butter over high heat, add pork loin, some salt and pepper, stir, brown for 10 minutes and transfer to a plate.
2. Add wine to the pan, bring to a boil over high heat and cook for 3 minutes.
3. Add stock, garlic, thyme spring, bay leaf, yellow onion and return meat to the pan, bring to a boil, cover, reduce heat to low, cook for 1 hour, strain liquid into another saucepan and transfer pork to a plate.

4. Put pearl onions in a small saucepan, add water to cover, bring to a boil over medium high heat, boil them for 5 minutes, drain, peel them and leave aside for now.
5. In a bowl, mix 2 tablespoons butter with flour and stir well. Add ½ cup of strained cooking liquid and whisk well.
6. Pour this into cooking liquid, bring to a simmer over medium heat and cook for 5 minutes. Add salt and pepper, chopped thyme, pork and pearl onions, cover and simmer for a few minutes.
7. Meanwhile, heat a pan with 1 tablespoon butter, add grapes, stir and cook them for 1-2 minutes. Divide pork meat on plates, drizzle the sauce all over and serve with onions and grapes on the side.

NUTRITION: Calories 320 Fat 31g Carbs 21g Protein 23g

# Pork and Chickpea Stew

Preparation time: 20 minutes

Cooking time: 8 hours

Servings: 4

INGREDIENTS:
- 2 tablespoons white flour
- ½ cup chicken stock
- 1 tablespoon ginger, grated
- 1 teaspoon coriander, ground
- 2 teaspoons cumin, ground
- Salt and black pepper to taste
- 2 and ½ pounds pork butt, cubed
- 28 ounces canned tomatoes, drained and chopped
- 4 ounces carrots, chopped
- 1 red onion cut in wedges
- 4 garlic cloves, minced
- ½ cup apricots, cut in quarters
- 1 cup couscous, cooked
- 15 ounces canned chickpeas, drained
- Cilantro, chopped for serving

DIRECTIONS:
1. Put stock in your slow cooker. Add flour, cumin, ginger, coriander, salt and pepper and stir. Add tomatoes, pork, carrots, garlic, onion and apricots, cover cooker and cook on Low for 7 hours and 50 minutes.
2. Add chickpeas and couscous, cover and cook for 10 more minutes. Divide on plates, sprinkle cilantro and serve right

away.
NUTRITION: Calories 216 Fat 31g Carbs 21g Protein 23g

# Pork and Greens Salad

Preparation time: 10 minutes

Cooking time:  15 minutes

Servings: 4

INGREDIENTS:
- 1-pound pork chops, boneless and cut into strips
- 8 ounces white mushrooms, sliced
- ½ cup Italian dressing
- 6 cups mixed salad greens
- 6 ounces jarred artichoke hearts, drained
- Salt and black pepper to the taste
- ½ cup basil, chopped
- 1 tablespoon olive oil

DIRECTIONS:
1. Heat a pan with the oil over medium-high heat, add the pork and brown for 5 minutes. Add the mushrooms, stir and sauté for 5 minutes more.
2. Add the dressing, artichokes, salad greens, salt, pepper and the basil, cook for 4-5 minutes, divide everything into bowls and serve.

NUTRITION: Calories 320 Fat 31g Carbs 21g Protein 23g

# Pork Strips and Rice

Preparation time: 10 minutes

Cooking time: 25 minutes

Servings: 4

INGREDIENTS:
- ½ pound pork loin, cut into strips
- Salt and black pepper to taste
- 2 tablespoons olive oil
- 2 carrots, chopped
- 1 red bell pepper, chopped
- 3 garlic cloves, minced
- 2 cups veggie stock
- 1 cup basmati rice
- ½ cup garbanzo beans
- 10 black olives, pitted and sliced
- 1 tablespoon parsley, chopped

DIRECTIONS:
1. Heat a pan with the oil over medium high heat. Add the pork fillets, stir, cook for 5 minutes and transfer them to a plate.
2. Add the carrots, bell pepper and the garlic, stir and cook for 5 more minutes.
3. Add the rice, the stock, beans and the olives, stir, cook for 14 minutes, divide between plates, sprinkle the parsley on top and serve.

NUTRITION: Calories 220 Fat 31g Carbs 21g Protein 23g

# Slow Cooked Mediterranean Pork

Preparation time: 20 hours and 10 minutes

Cooking time: 8 hours

Servings: 6

INGREDIENTS:
- 3 pounds pork shoulder - boneless
- ¼ cup olive oil
- 2 teaspoons oregano, dried
- ¼ cup lemon juice
- 2 teaspoons mustard
- 2 teaspoons mint, chopped
- 3 garlic cloves, minced
- 2 teaspoons pesto sauce
- Salt and black pepper to taste

DIRECTIONS:
1. In a bowl, mix olive oil with lemon juice, oregano, mint, mustard, garlic, pesto, salt and pepper then whisk well.
2. Rub pork with marinade, cover and keep in a cold place for 10 hours. Flip pork shoulder and leave aside for 10 more hours.
3. Transfer to your slow cooker along with the marinade juices, cover and cook on low for 8 hours. Uncover, slice, divide between plates and serve.

NUTRITION: Calories 320 Fat 31g Carbs 21g Protein 23g

# Pork and Bean Stew

Preparation time: 20 minutes

Cooking time: 4 hours

Servings: 4

INGREDIENTS:
- 2 pounds pork neck
- 1 tablespoon white flour
- 1 and ½ tablespoons olive oil
- 2 eggplants, chopped
- 1 brown onion, chopped
- 1 red bell pepper, chopped
- 3 garlic cloves, minced
- 1 tablespoon thyme, dried
- 2 teaspoons sage, dried
- 4 ounces canned white beans, drained
- 1 cup chicken stock
- 12 ounces zucchinis, chopped
- Salt and pepper to taste
- 2 tablespoons tomato paste

DIRECTIONS:
1. In a bowl, mix flour with salt, pepper, pork neck and toss. Heat a pan with 2 teaspoons oil over medium high heat, add pork and cook for 3 minutes on each side.
2. Transfer pork to a slow cooker and leave aside. Heat the remaining oil in the same pan over medium heat, add eggplant, onion, bell pepper, thyme, sage and garlic, stir and cook for 5 minutes.
3. Add reserved flour, stir and cook for 1 more minute. Add to pork, then add beans,

stock, tomato paste and zucchinis. Cover and cook on high for 4 hours. Uncover, transfer to plates and serve.

NUTRITION: Calories: 310 fat 31g carbs 21g protein 23g

www.ingramcontent.com/pod-product-compliance
Lightning Source LLC
Chambersburg PA
CBHW050750030426
42336CB00012B/1740